MW00939693

THE MAGNET® MODEL
COMPONENTS AND
SOURCES OF EVIDENCE
MAGNET RECOGNITION PROGRAM®

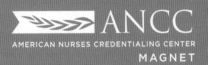

ANCC
AMERICAN NURSES CREDENTIALING CENTER
MAGNET

Innovate. Involve. Inspire.

AMERICAN NURSES CREDENTIALING CENTER

The American Nurses Credentialing Center (ANCC) provides people and organizations in the nursing profession with the tools they need on their journey to excellence. ANCC recognizes healthcare organizations for nursing excellence through the Magnet Recognition Program®. ANCC is the largest and most prestigious nurse-credentialing organization in the United States.

Commission on Magnet® Recognition

The ANCC's Commission on Magnet® Recognition is a voluntary governing body that oversees the Magnet Recognition Program. Commission members are appointed by the ANCC's board of directors and are representatives from various sectors of the nursing community, which includes nursing executive leaders, nurse managers, staff nurses, long-term-care nurses, and advanced practice registered nurses. One commission member represents public consumers. The Commission on Magnet Recognition makes the final determination of award designation.

Magnet® Appraisers

Appraisers are leading expert nurses with demonstrated expertise and experience in various organizational and specialty backgrounds relevant to the Magnet Recognition Program. They evaluate applicant documents, conduct site visits, and prepare the final report to the Commission on Magnet Recognition. Appraisers are selected through a competitive application process. All appraisers undergo intensive training on the interpretation and evaluation of Sources of Evidence for the Magnet appraisal process before being assigned to any appraiser team.

Magnet® Program Office

The ANCC's Magnet program office staff manages and coordinates all aspects of the application and appraisal process. Contact information is available at www.nursecredentialing.org/magnet/magnetcontacts.

Published by American Nurses Credentialing Center
8515 Georgia Avenue, Suite 400
Silver Spring, MD 20910-3492

Copyright ©2013 by American Nurses Credentialing Center, Silver Spring, MD
2014 edition. ISBN-13: 978-1492358787

A subsidiary of the American Nurses Association

Disclaimers:

Please note: this is an abridged version of the *2014 Magnet® Application Manual*. If your organization is considering pursuing Magnet recognition, the 2014 edition of the *Magnet Manual* is essential for understanding the full scope of application requirements. It is the only authorized publication that provides detailed information on the instructions and process for documentation submission. To order a copy of the *2014 Magnet® Application Manual*, or obtain additional information about the Magnet Recognition Program, visit our website at www.nursecredentialing.org/magnet.

The Magnet® Vision

Magnet® organizations will serve as the fount of knowledge and expertise for the delivery of nursing care globally. They will be solidly grounded in core Magnet principles, flexible, and constantly striving for discovery and innovation. They will lead the reformation of health care; the discipline of nursing; and care of the patient, family, and community.

The Commission on Magnet Recognition, 2008

THE MAGNET® MODEL COMPONENTS AND SOURCES OF EVIDENCE

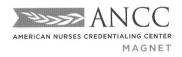

ANCC
AMERICAN NURSES CREDENTIALING CENTER
MAGNET

Table of Contents

NOTE:

While this abridged version provides valuable information, if you are on the Journey to Magnet Excellence® or considering applying for Magnet® status, you need to refer to the *2014 Magnet® Application Manual* for complete requirements and guidance.

Introduction

ANCC's Magnet® designation is the highest and most prestigious credential a healthcare organization can achieve for nursing excellence and quality patient care. This performance-driven credential brings wide-ranging benefits, including improved safety, nurse satisfaction and retention, reduced costs, and superior patient outcomes. In fact, the application and peer review process itself often provides valuable feedback and improvement opportunities.

Magnet is raising the bar for nursing care delivery, new nursing knowledge, and evidence-based clinical quality in healthcare organizations around the world. As we look forward, we see a growing community of Magnet hospitals and a new generation of global gold standards that guide quality patient care. In addition, an increased focus on outcomes will help all organizations demonstrate the value nursing brings to the patient, the organization, and the community.

The Magnet® Model Components and Sources of Evidence is an abridged version of the *2014 Magnet® Application Manual* and includes key program elements: the Magnet Model and its components, the sources of evidence used in the appraisal process, and references and the glossary.

We hope this guide serves as a resource for those who seek to understand the important variables that interact to create a culture of excellence, and the role nurses play in impacting those outcomes.

Patricia Reid Ponte, DNSc, RN, NEA-BC, FAAN
Chair, Commission on Magnet Recognition

Karen Drenkard, PhD, RN, NEA-BC, FAAN
Executive Director, American Nurses Credentialing Center

Chapter 1

THE MAGNET® MODEL

The Forces of Magnetism that were identified more than 25 years ago have remained remarkably stable—a testament to their enduring value. The Magnet Recognition Program® evolved over time in response to changes in the healthcare environment.

Statistical Foundation—the Empirical Model

In 2007, the American Nurses Credentialing Center commissioned a statistical analysis of final appraisal scores for applicants under the 2005 *Magnet Recognition Program Application Manual* (ANCC, 2004). The project goal was to examine the relationships among the Forces of Magnetism by investigating alternative frameworks for structuring the Sources of Evidence and to inform development of the new Magnet Model. This newly emerged Magnet Model would provide a new perspective on the Sources of Evidence and how they interplay to create a work environment that supports excellence in nursing practice.

Through the use of a combination of factor analysis, cluster analysis, and multidimensional scaling, final Sources of Evidence scores were examined to determine how they might be organized based solely on their empirical properties. The results suggested an alternative framework for grouping the Sources of Evidence, collapsing them into fewer domains than the 14 Forces of Magnetism. The empiric model yielded from this analysis informed the conceptual development of the new Magnet Model.

The Magnet Model

In 2007, with input from a broad representation of stakeholders, the Commission on Magnet Recognition developed a model for Magnet that reflected current research on organizational behavior. This Magnet Model guides the transition of Magnet principles to focus healthcare organizations on achieving superior performance as evidenced by outcomes. Evidence-based practice, innovation, evolving technology, and patient partnerships are evident in the Magnet Model (see **Figure 1**).

FIGURE 1. MAGNET MODEL

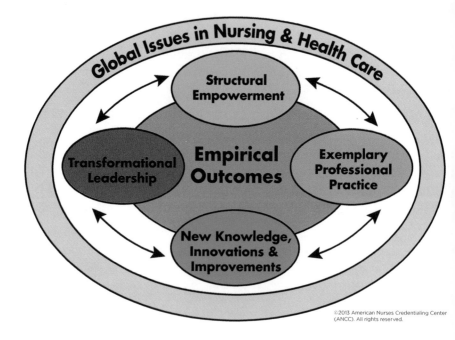

Focus on Outcomes

A fundamental shift occurred with the 2008 introduction of the Magnet Model to incorporate outcomes.

Previous *Magnet Application Manuals* emphasized structure and process. Although structure and process create the infrastructure for excellence, the outcomes of that infrastructure are essential to a culture of excellence and innovation.

Simple definitions are set forth to differentiate among structure, process, and outcomes:

▸ **Structure** is defined as the characteristics of the organization and the healthcare system, including leadership, availability of resources, and professional practice models.

▸ **Process** is defined as the actions involving the delivery of nursing and healthcare services to patients, including practices that are safe and ethical, autonomous, and evidence-based, with efforts focused on quality improvement.

▸ **Outcomes** are defined as quantitative and qualitative evidence related to the impact of structure and process on the patient, the nursing workforce, the organization, and the consumer. These outcomes are dynamic and measurable and may be reported at an individual unit, department, population, or organizational level.

Empirical Outcomes (EOs) are required throughout the Magnet Model components and are denoted by EO for the outcome Sources of Evidence. Requirements for narratives, graphs, tables, and formatting for all EOs are found in the Empirical Outcomes section of the *2014 Magnet® Application Manual.*

TABLE 1. FORCES OF MAGNETISM AND DERIVATION OF THE MAGNET MODEL

Forces of Magnetism	Empirical Domains of Evidence	Magnet Model Components
1. Quality of Nursing Leadership 3. Management Style	Leadership	Transformational Leadership
2. Organizational Structure 4. Personnel Policies and Programs 10. Community and the Healthcare Organization 12. Image of Nursing 14. Professional Development	Resource Utilization and Development	Structural Empowerment
5. Professional Models of Care 8. Consultation and Resources 9. Autonomy 11. Nurses as Teachers 13. Interdisciplinary (Interprofessional) Relationships 6. Quality of Care: Ethics, Patient Safety, and Quality Infrastructure 7. Quality Improvement	Professional Practice Model Safe and Ethical Practice Autonomous Practice Quality Processes	Exemplary Professional Practice
6. Quality of Care: Research- and Evidence-Based Practice 7. Quality Improvement	Research	New Knowledge, Innovations & Improvements
6. Quality of Care	Outcomes	Empirical Quality Outcomes

Chapter 2

MAGNET® MODEL COMPONENTS AND SOURCES OF EVIDENCE

This section describes the expectations for each of the five Magnet Model components and lists the Magnet® program requirements as Sources of Evidence. **Table 2** depicts the labeling convention used to refer to the Sources of Evidence by Magnet Model component (e.g., TL2, TL1EO). Note that the empirical outcome standards are embedded as part of the other four Magnet Model components. The Sources of Evidence (i.e., TL, SE, EP, NK) are further subcategorized for easy understanding (e.g., Strategic Planning, Advocacy and Influence, Visibility and Accessibility).

TABLE 2. REFERENCE LABELS OF THE SOURCES OF EVIDENCE

Label for Source of Evidence (SOE)	Model Component	Standard Number	SOE With Empirical Outcome
TL	Transformational Leadership	TL2, TL4, etc.	TL1EO, TL3EO, etc.
SE	Structural Empowerment	SE6, SE7, etc.	SE1EO, SE2EO, etc.
EP	Exemplary Professional Practice	EP1, EP4, etc.	EP2EO, EP3EO, etc.
NK	New Knowledge, Innovations & Improvements	NK2, NK3, etc.	NK1EO, NK4EO, etc.
EO	Empirical Outcomes		

I. TRANSFORMATIONAL LEADERSHIP (TL)

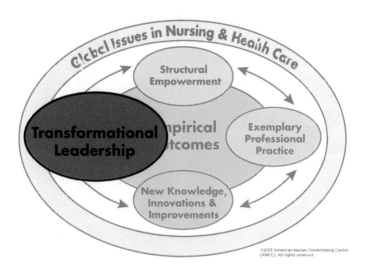

Forces of Magnetism:

▸ Quality of Nursing

▸ Management Style

The chief nursing officer (CNO) in a Magnet-recognized organization is a knowledgeable, transformational leader who develops a strong vision and well-articulated philosophy, a professional practice model, and strategic and quality plans in leading nursing services. The transformational CNO communicates expectations, develops leaders, and evolves the organization to meet current and anticipated needs and strategic priorities. Nursing leaders at all levels of the organization demonstrate advocacy and support on behalf of staff and patients.

The CNO must be strategically positioned within the organization to effectively influence other executive stakeholders, including the board of directors/trustees. Strategic positioning is imperative to achieve the level of influence required to lead others, both operationally and during periods of change management, because of internal or external factors. Executive-level nursing leaders serve at the highest level of the organization, with the CNO typically reporting to the chief executive officer.

Nursing's mission, vision, values, and strategic plan must align with the organization's priorities to improve the organization's performance. Wherever nursing is practiced, the CNO must develop structures, processes, and expectations for clinical nurse input and involvement throughout the organization. Mechanisms must be implemented for evidence-based practice to evolve and for innovation to flourish. The CNO should be seen as an executive leader and a nursing advocate and perceived as leading nursing practice and patient care. The CNO should be visible and accessible and should communicate effectively in an environment of mutual respect. As a result, nurses throughout the organization should perceive that their voices are heard, their input is valued, and their practice is supported.

Sources of Evidence

STRATEGIC PLANNING

TL1EO **Nursing's mission, vision, values, and strategic plan align with the organization's priorities to improve the organization's performance.**

> ▸ Provide one example, with supporting evidence, of an initiative identified in the nursing strategic plan that resulted in an improvement in the nurse practice environment. Supporting evidence must be submitted in the form of a graph with a data table that clearly displays the data.

> AND

> ▸ Provide one example, with supporting evidence, of an initiative identified in the nursing strategic plan that resulted in an improvement due to a change in clinical practice. Supporting evidence must be submitted in the form of a graph with a data table that clearly displays the data.

TL2 **Nurse leaders and clinical nurses advocate for resources to support nursing unit and organizational goals.**

▸ Provide one example, with supporting evidence, of a nurse leader's advocacy that resulted in the allocation of resources to support an organizational goal.

AND

▸ Provide one example, with supporting evidence, of a clinical nurse's (or clinical nurses') advocacy that resulted in the allocation of resources to support a nursing unit goal.

ADVOCACY AND INFLUENCE

TL3EO **The CNO influences organization-wide change beyond the scope of nursing.**

▸ Provide one example, with supporting evidence, of a CNO-influenced positive change that had organization-wide impact beyond the scope of nursing services. Supporting evidence must be submitted in the form of a graph with a data table that clearly displays the data.

TL4 **The CNO is a strategic partner in the organization's decision-making.**

▸ Provide one example, with supporting evidence, of the CNO's involvement in the organization's decision-making (not involving technology).

AND

▸ Provide one example, with supporting evidence, of the CNO's involvement in the organization's technology decision-making.

TL5   **Nurse leaders lead effectively through change.**

- ▸ Provide one example, with supporting evidence, of the strategies used by nurse leaders to successfully guide nurses through unplanned change.

AND

- ▸ Provide one example, with supporting evidence, of the strategies used by nurse leaders to successfully guide nurses through planned change.

TL6   **The CNO advocates for organizational support of ongoing leadership development for all nurses, with a focus on mentoring and succession planning.**

- ▸ Provide one example, with supporting evidence, of each of the following activities:

  - ▸▸ Mentoring or succession planning activities for clinical nurses

  AND

  - ▸▸ Mentoring or succession planning activities for nurse managers

  AND

  - ▸▸ Mentoring or succession planning activities for nurse leaders (exclusive of nurse managers)

  AND

  - ▸▸ Mentoring or succession planning activities for the chief nursing officer

TL7 **Nurse leaders, with clinical nurse input, use trended data to acquire necessary resources to support the care delivery system(s).**

  ▸ Provide one example, with supporting evidence, where a nurse leader, with clinical nurse input, used trended data to acquire necessary resources to support the care delivery system(s).

VISIBILITY, ACCESSIBILITY, AND COMMUNICATION

TL8 **The CNO uses various methods to communicate, be visible, and be accessible to nurses throughout the organization. Choose two of the three below:**

  ▸ Provide one example, with supporting evidence, of communication between the clinical nurse(s) and the CNO that led to a change in the nurse practice environment.

  OR

  ▸ Provide one example, with supporting evidence, of communication between the clinical nurse(s) and the CNO that led to a change in the patient experience.

  OR

  ▸ Provide one example, with supporting evidence, of communication between the clinical nurse(s) and the CNO that influenced a change in nursing practice.

TL9EO **Nurse leaders (exclusive of the CNO) use input from clinical nurses to influence change in the organization. Choose two of the three below (examples must be different from those provided in TL8):**

▸ Provide one example, with supporting evidence, of a change in the nurse practice environment that was influenced by the clinical nurses' communication with a nurse leader. Supporting evidence must be submitted in the form of a graph with a data table that clearly displays the data.

OR

▸ Provide one example, with supporting evidence, of a change in the patient experience that was influenced by the clinical nurses' communication with a nurse leader. Supporting evidence must be submitted in the form of a graph with a data table that clearly displays the data.

OR

▸ Provide one example, with supporting evidence, of a change in nursing practice that was influenced by the clinical nurses' communication with a nurse leader. Supporting evidence must be submitted in the form of a graph with a data table that clearly displays the data.

II. STRUCTURAL EMPOWERMENT (SE)

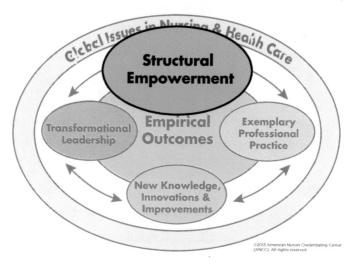

©2013 American Nurses Credentialing Center (ANCC). All rights reserved.

Forces of Magnetism:

▶ Organizational Structure

▶ Personnel Policies and Programs

▶ Community and the Healthcare Organization

▶ Image of Nursing

▶ Professional Development

 International Equivalent, see Appendix F in the *2014 Magnet® Application Manual*

Magnet structural environments are generally flat, flexible, and decentralized. Nurses throughout the organization are involved in shared-governance and decision-making structures and processes that establish standards of practice and address opportunities for improvement.

The flow of information and decision-making is multidirectional among professional nurses at the bedside, leadership, interprofessional teams, and the chief nursing officer. The CNO serves on the highest-level decision-making bodies, such as councils, committees, and task forces that influence the organization's mission, vision, values, and strategic goals. In addition, nurse leaders throughout the organization serve on decision-making bodies that address excellence in patient care and the safe, efficient, and effective operation of the organization.

Magnet-recognized organizations promote and develop strong partnerships with community organizations to improve patient outcomes and advance the health of the communities they serve. In addition, Magnet nurses support organizational goals, advance the nursing profession, and enhance professional development by extending their influence to professional and community groups. Nursing contributions to improved community healthcare services are acknowledged by Magnet-recognized organizations in substantive ways that enhance and support the value and image of nursing within the organization and the community at large.

Magnet-recognized organizations use multiple strategies to create structures and processes that support a lifelong learning culture that includes professional collaboration and the promotion of role development, academic achievement, and career advancement.

Sources of Evidence

PROFESSIONAL DEVELOPMENT

SE1EO **Clinical nurses are involved in interprofessional decision-making groups at the organizational level.** (Examples include, but are not limited to, organizational quality councils, budget review committees, equipment selection committees, mortality and morbidity committees, pharmacy and therapeutics committees, blood utilization committees, safety committees, and bioethics committees.)

> ▹ Provide two examples, with supporting evidence, of improvements resulting from the contributions of clinical nurses in interprofessional decision-making groups at the organizational level. Supporting evidence must be submitted in the form of a graph with a data table that clearly displays the data.

The healthcare organization supports nurses' participation in local, regional, national, or international professional organizations.

▸ Provide two examples, with supporting evidence, of improvements resulting from a change in nursing practice that occurred because of clinical nurse involvement in a professional organization. Supporting evidence must be submitted in the form of a graph with a data table that clearly displays the data.

COMMITMENT TO PROFESSIONAL DEVELOPMENT

SE3EO **The organization supports nurses' continuous professional development.**

IE

▸ Provide one example, with supporting evidence, illustrating that the organization has met a targeted goal for improvement in professional nursing certification. Supporting evidence must be submitted in the form of a graph with a data table that clearly displays the data.

AND

▸ Provide one example, with supporting evidence, illustrating that nursing has met a targeted goal for improvement in professional nursing certification by unit or division (e.g., cardiac-vascular, gerontological, medical-surgical, nursing informatics, pediatrics, psychiatric–mental health). Supporting evidence must be submitted in the form of a graph with a data table that clearly displays the data.

SE4EO **Nurses participate in professional development activities designed to improve their knowledge, skills, and/or practices in the workplace. Professional development activities are designed to improve the professional practice of nursing or patient outcomes, or both. May include interprofessional activities.**

Does not include orientation-related education.

▸ Provide one example, with supporting evidence, of nurses' participation in a professional development activity that demonstrated an improvement in knowledge, skills, and/or practices for professional registered nurses. Supporting evidence must be submitted in the form of a graph with a data table that clearly displays the data.

AND

▸ Provide one example, with supporting evidence, of nurses' participation in a professional development activity that was associated with an improvement in a patient care outcome. Supporting evidence must be submitted in the form of a graph with a data table that clearly displays the data.

SE5 **Nursing education opportunities are provided for those interested in a nursing career.**

▸ Provide one example, with supporting evidence, of a career development opportunity provided by the organization for non-nurse employees or members of the community interested in becoming a registered nurse. This example may include community partnership activities.

TEACHING AND ROLE DEVELOPMENT

SE6   **The organization provides opportunities to improve nurses' expertise in effectively teaching a patient or family.**

> ▸ Provide one example, with supporting evidence, of an educational activity provided by the organization focused on improving nurses' expertise in teaching a patient or family.

SE7   **The organization facilitates the effective transition of registered nurses and advanced practice registered nurses into the work environment. Choose two of the four below:**

> ▸ Provide one example, with supporting evidence, of how the organization facilitates effective transition of new graduate nurses into the nurse practice environment. Describe how the transition process is evaluated for effectiveness.

OR

> ▸ Provide one example, with supporting evidence, of how the organization facilitates effective transition of newly hired experienced nurses into the nurse practice environment. Describe how the transition process is evaluated for effectiveness.

OR

> ▸ Provide one example, with supporting evidence, of how the organization facilitates effective transition of nurses transferring within the organization from one specialty care area to a different specialty care area. Describe how the transition process is evaluated for effectiveness.

OR

> ▸ Provide one example, with supporting evidence, of how the organization facilitates effective transition of advanced practice registered nurses into practice within the organization. Describe how the transition process is evaluated for effectiveness.

SE8   **The organization provides educational activities to improve the nurse's expertise as a preceptor.**

> ▸ Describe the organization's preceptor educational program(s) and how each program is evaluated on an ongoing basis. Provide supporting evidence.

COMMITMENT TO COMMUNITY INVOLVEMENT

SE9   **The organization supports nurses' participation in community healthcare outreach.**

> ▸ Provide one example, with supporting evidence, of organizational support for clinical nurse involvement in community healthcare outreach.

AND

> ▸ Provide one example, with supporting evidence, of organizational support for nurse leader involvement in community healthcare outreach.

SE10EO **Nurses participate in the assessment and prioritization of the healthcare needs of the community.**

> ▸ Provide one example, with supporting evidence, of an improvement in an identified healthcare need that was associated with nurses' partnership with the community. Supporting evidence must be submitted in the form of a graph with a data table that clearly displays the data.

RECOGNITION OF NURSING

SE11   **Nurses are recognized for their contributions in addressing the strategic priorities of the organization.**

> ▸ Provide one example, with supporting evidence, of recognition of a clinical nurse for his or her contribution(s) in addressing the strategic priorities of the organization.

AND

> ▸ Provide one example, with supporting evidence, of recognition of a group of nurses for their contribution(s) in addressing the strategic priorities of the organization.

III. EXEMPLARY PROFESSIONAL PRACTICE (EP)

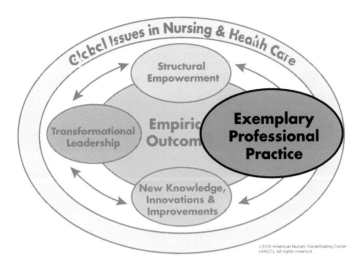

Forces of Magnetism:

▶ Professional Models of Care

▶ Consultation and Resources

▶ Autonomy

▶ Nurses as Teachers

▶ Interdisciplinary (Interprofessional) Relationships

▶ Quality of Care: Ethics, Patient Safety, and Quality Infrastructure

▶ Quality Improvement

 International Equivalent, see Appendix F in the *2014 Magnet® Application Manual*

A professional practice model is the overarching conceptual framework for nurses, nursing care, and interprofessional patient care. It is a schematic description of a system, theory, or phenomenon that depicts how nurses

practice, collaborate, communicate, and develop professionally to provide the highest-quality care for those served by the organization (e.g., patients, families, communities). The professional practice model illustrates the alignment and integration of nursing practice with the mission, vision, values, and philosophy that nursing has adopted. At the organizational level, nurse leaders ensure that care is patient/family centered. Magnet-recognized organizations take the lead in research efforts to create and test models that promote the professional practice of nurses.

The care delivery system is integrated within the professional practice model and promotes continuous, consistent, efficient, and accountable delivery of nursing care. The care delivery system is adapted to meet evidence-based practice standards, national patient safety goals, affordable and value-based outcomes, and regulatory requirements. It describes the manner in which care is delivered, the skill set required, the context of care, and the expected outcomes of care. Nurses create patient care delivery systems that delineate the nurses' shared authority and accountability for evidence-based nursing practice, clinical decision-making and outcomes, performance improvement initiatives, and staffing and scheduling processes.

Exemplary professional practice in Magnet-recognized organizations is evidenced by effective and efficient care services, interprofessional collaboration, and high-quality patient outcomes. Magnet nurses partner with patients, families, support systems, and interprofessional teams to positively impact patient care and outcomes. Interprofessional team members include but are not limited to personnel from medicine, pharmacy, nutrition, rehabilitation, social work, psychology, and other professions that collaborate to ensure a comprehensive plan of care. Collegial working relationships within and among the disciplines are valued and promoted by the organization's leadership and its employees. Mutual respect is based on the premise that all members of the healthcare team make essential and meaningful contributions to the achievement of clinical outcomes. Conflict management strategies are in place and are used effectively.

The autonomous nurse provides care based on the unique needs and attributes of the patient and his or her family and/or support system. The knowledge, skills, and resources that have been identified by the nursing staff as necessary to practice are the foundation for the care delivery system; therefore, they are consistently available in the practice environment. Competency assessment and peer evaluation ensure that nurses deliver safe, ethical, and evidence-based nursing care.

Workplace advocacy initiatives include but are not limited to addressing ethical issues, patient rights, privacy, security, and patient and staff confidentiality. Magnet-recognized organizations embrace a culture that empowers nurses and other staff to identify and bring forth concerns without fear of retribution. Attention is given to achieving equity of care and equity in the workplace environment.

The achievement of exemplary professional practice is grounded in a culture of safety, quality monitoring, and quality improvement. Nurses collaborate with other disciplines to ensure that care is comprehensive, coordinated, and monitored for effectiveness through the quality improvement model. Nurses participate in safety initiatives that incorporate national best practices. Sufficient resources are available to respond to safety initiatives and quality improvements for patients and employees.

Nurses at all levels analyze data and use national benchmarks to gain a comparative perspective about their performance and the care patients receive. Action plans are developed that lead to systematic improvements over time. Magnet organization data demonstrate outcome measures that generally outperform the benchmark statistic of the national database used in patient- and nurse-sensitive indicators.

PROFESSIONAL PRACTICE MODEL

EP1 **Clinical nurses are involved in the development, implementation, and evaluation of the professional practice model.**

> ▸ **New applicants:** Provide a description, with supporting evidence, of the development of the nursing professional practice model and how clinical nurses were involved.

> ▸ **Redesignating applicants:** Provide a description, with supporting evidence, of the ongoing evaluation of the nursing professional practice model and how clinical nurses are involved.

EP2EO **Clinical nurses are involved in the development, implementation, and evaluation of the professional practice model.**

> ▸ Provide one example, with supporting evidence, of an improvement resulting from a change in clinical practice that occurred because of clinical nurses' involvement in the implementation or evaluation of the professional practice model. Supporting evidence must be submitted in the form of a graph with a data table that clearly displays the data.

EP3EO **Unit or clinic level nurse (RN) satisfaction data outperform the mean or median of the national database used.**

IE

Note: Benchmark used must be one to which the organization contributes data.

> ▸ Provide unit-based, national benchmarked nurse (RN) satisfaction data from the most recent survey administered within the previous 30 months before documentation submission. Example shown in **Figure 3**.

▸ **This SOE becomes effective April 1, 2016.** Until that time, the 2008 EP3EO is in effect. 2008 *Application Manual* EP3EO: Nurse satisfaction or engagement data aggregated at the organizational, clinical groups of like-units or unit level outperform the mean, median, or other benchmark statistic of the national database used. Submit data for the most recent nurse satisfaction survey within the previous 30 months before documentation submission. Include participation rates, analysis, and evaluation of the data.

Nurse (RN) satisfaction survey must include questions related to the following seven categories. Data must be submitted on your choice of four of the seven categories.

1. Autonomy
2. Professional development (education, resources, etc.)
3. Leadership access and responsiveness (includes nursing administration/CNO)
4. Interprofessional relationships (includes all disciplines)
5. Fundamentals of quality nursing care
6. Adequacy of resources and staffing
7. RN-to-RN teamwork and collaboration

CARE DELIVERY SYSTEM(S)

EP4   **Nurses create partnerships with patients and families to establish goals and plans for delivery of patient-centered care.**

▸ Provide one example, with supporting evidence, of nurses partnering with patients and families to develop an individualized plan of care based on the unique needs of the patient.

AND

▸ Provide one example, with supporting evidence, of nurses partnering with patients and families to improve systems of care at the unit, service line, or organizational level.

EP5   **Nurses are involved in interprofessional collaborative practice within the care delivery system to ensure care coordination and continuity of care.**

▸ Provide two examples, with supporting evidence, of nurses' involvement in interprofessional collaborative practice that ensures care coordination and continuity of patient care.

EP6   **Nurses incorporate regulatory and specialty standards/ guidelines into the development and implementation of the care delivery system.**

▸ Provide one example, with supporting evidence, of nurses incorporating specialty standards/guidelines into the delivery of care.

EP7EO **Nurses systematically evaluate professional organizations' standards of practice, incorporating them into the organization's professional practice model and care delivery system.**

> ▸ Provide one example, with supporting evidence, of an improvement resulting from a change in clinical practice due to the application of a professional organizations' standards of nursing practice. The example provided may be at the unit, division, or organizational level. Supporting evidence must be submitted in the form of a graph with a data table that clearly displays the data.

EP8EO **Nurses use internal and external experts to improve the clinical practice setting.**

> ▸ Provide one example, with supporting evidence, of an improvement that occurred due to a change in clinical practice setting resulting from the use of internal experts. Supporting evidence must be submitted in the form of a graph with a data table that clearly displays the data.

> OR

> ▸ Provide one example, with supporting evidence, of an improvement that occurred due to a change in the clinical practice setting resulting from the use of external experts. Supporting evidence must be submitted in the form of a graph with a data table that clearly displays the data.

STAFFING, SCHEDULING, AND BUDGETING PROCESSES

EP9 **Nurses are involved in staffing and scheduling based on established guidelines, such as ANA's *Principles for Nurse Staffing*, to ensure that RN assignments meet the needs of the patient population.**

> ▸ Provide two examples, with supporting evidence, from different practice settings when input from clinical nurses was used to modify RN staffing assignments and/or adjust the schedule to compensate for a change in patient acuity, patient population, resources, or redesign of care.

EP10   **Nurses use trended data in the budgeting process, with clinical nurse input, to redistribute existing nursing resources or obtain additional nursing resources.**

> ▸ Provide two examples with supporting evidence from different practice settings where trended data was used during the budget process, with clinical nurse input, to assess actual-to-budget performance to redistribute existing nursing resources or to acquire additional nursing resources. Trended data must be presented.

EP11EO   **Nurses participate in recruitment and retention assessment and planning activities.**

> ▸ Provide one example, with supporting evidence, of clinical nurses' participation in nursing recruitment activities and the impact on vacancy rates. Supporting evidence must be submitted in the form of a graph with a data table that clearly displays the data.

OR

> ▸ Provide one example, with supporting evidence, of clinical nurses' participation in nursing retention activities and the impact on turnover rates. Supporting evidence must be submitted in the form of a graph with a data table that clearly displays the data.

INTERPROFESSIONAL CARE

EP12   **Nurses assume leadership roles in collaborative interprofessional activities to improve the quality of care.**

> ▸ Provide one example, with supporting evidence, of a nurse-led (or nurse co-led) collaborative interprofessional quality improvement activity.

EP13EO **Nurses participate in interprofessional groups that implement and evaluate coordinated patient education activities.**

> ▸ Provide one example, with supporting evidence, of an interprofessional patient education activity that was associated with an improved patient outcome. Supporting evidence must be submitted in the form of a graph with a data table that clearly displays the data.

ACCOUNTABILITY, COMPETENCE, AND AUTONOMY

EP14 **Resources, such as professional literature, are readily available to support decision-making in autonomous nursing practice.**

> ▸ Provide two examples, with supporting evidence, of how resources are used to support evidence-based clinical decision-making in autonomous nursing practice.

EP15 **Nurses at all levels engage in periodic formal performance reviews that include a self-appraisal and peer feedback process for assurance of competence and continuous professional development.**

> ▸ Provide one example, with supporting evidence, of clinical nurses using periodic formal performance review that includes a self-appraisal and peer feedback process to enhance competence or professional development.
>
> AND
>
> ▸ Provide one example, with supporting evidence, of nurse leaders using periodic formal performance review that includes a self-appraisal and peer feedback process to enhance competence or professional development.
>
> *Note: The CNO and nurse educators are included in nurse leaders.*

EP 16　**Nurse autonomy is supported and promoted through the organization's governance structure for shared decision-making.**

▸ Provide one example, with supporting evidence, of clinical autonomy that demonstrates the authority and freedom of nurses to make nursing care decisions (within the full scope of their practice) in the clinical care of patients.

AND

▸ Provide one example, with supporting evidence, of organizational autonomy that demonstrates the authority and freedom of nurses to be involved in broader unit, service line, organization, or system decision-making processes pertaining to patient care, policies and procedures, or work environment.

ETHICS, PRIVACY, SECURITY, AND CONFIDENTIALITY

EP17　**Nurses use available resources to address ethical issues related to clinical practice and organizational ethical situations.**

▸ Provide one example, with supporting evidence, of nurses using available resources to address ethical issues related to clinical practice.

OR

▸ Provide one example, with supporting evidence, of nurses using available resources to address an organizational ethical issue.

CULTURE OF SAFETY

EP18EO　**Workplace safety for nurses is evaluated and improved.**

▸ Provide two examples, with supporting evidence, of improved workplace safety for nurses resulting from the safety strategy of the organization. Supporting evidence must be submitted in the form of a graph with a data table that clearly displays the data.

EP19EO **Nurses are involved in the facility- or system-wide approach focused on proactive risk assessment and error management.**

▸ Provide one example, with supporting evidence, of an improvement in patient safety that resulted from nurses' involvement in facility- or system-wide proactive risk assessment or error management. Supporting evidence must be submitted in the form of a graph with a data table that clearly displays the data.

EP20EO **Clinical nurses are involved in the review, action planning, and evaluation of patient safety data at the unit level.**

▸ Provide two examples, with supporting evidence, of an improvement in patient safety that resulted from clinical nurses' involvement in the evaluation of patient safety data at the unit level. Supporting evidence must be submitted in the form of a graph with a data table that clearly displays the data.

EP21EO **Nurses are involved in implementing and evaluating national or international patient safety goals.**

▸ Provide one example, with supporting evidence, of nurses' involvement in activities that address national or international patient safety goals that led to an improvement in patient safety outcomes. Supporting evidence must be submitted in the form of a graph with a data table that clearly displays the data.

EP22EO Unit- or clinic-level nurse-sensitive clinical indicator data outperform the mean or median of the national database used.

IE

For an acute care organization with or without ambulatory/outpatient services, six nurse-sensitive clinical indicators are required. The required indicators for all acute care organizations include falls with injury, hospital-acquired pressure ulcers stages 2 and above, central line-associated bloodstream infection, and catheter-associated urinary tract infection. For organizations with ambulatory/outpatient services only, two nurse-sensitive clinical indicators are required.

Organizations seeking Magnet designation must submit the following:

▸ Provide nationally benchmarked unit- or clinic-level nurse-sensitive clinical indicator data using tables and graphs to display 8 quarters of data for the 30 months before documentation submission.

▸ Use national databases when available. If a national database is not available, the organization must demonstrate that internal benchmarks are based on professional standards, literature review, or internal trended data, or all three.

For complete information about clinical indicator requirements, see the comprehensive information in the *2014 Magnet® Application Manual*.

See *Addendum* on page 109 in the *2014 Magnet® Application Manual* for requirements ONLY for international and speciality organizations, and Core Measure Sets.

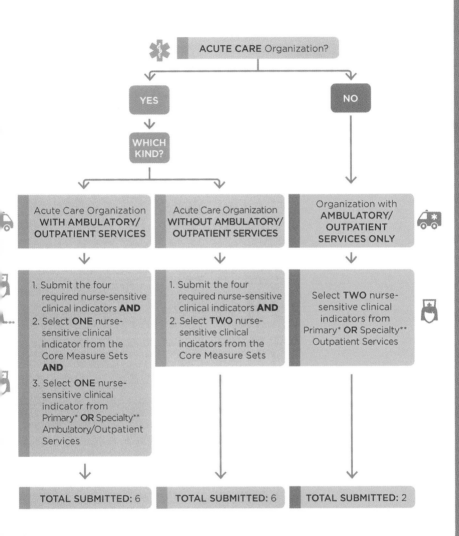

ACUTE CARE Organization?

YES → **NO**

WHICH KIND?

Acute Care Organization **WITH AMBULATORY/ OUTPATIENT SERVICES**	Acute Care Organization **WITHOUT AMBULATORY/ OUTPATIENT SERVICES**	Organization with **AMBULATORY/ OUTPATIENT SERVICES ONLY**
1. Submit the four required nurse-sensitive clinical indicators **AND** 2. Select **ONE** nurse-sensitive clinical indicator from the Core Measure Sets **AND** 3. Select **ONE** nurse-sensitive clinical indicator from Primary* **OR** Specialty** Ambulatory/Outpatient Services	1. Submit the four required nurse-sensitive clinical indicators **AND** 2. Select **TWO** nurse-sensitive clinical indicators from the Core Measure Sets	Select **TWO** nurse-sensitive clinical indicators from Primary* **OR** Specialty** Outpatient Services
TOTAL SUBMITTED: 6	**TOTAL SUBMITTED:** 6	**TOTAL SUBMITTED:** 2

*Primary: Examples include, but are not limited to, readmission rates related to diabetes, CHF, COPD, asthma, pain management; unplanned admissions to higher level of care.

**Specialty: Examples include, but are not limited to, unplanned admissions, pain management, medication errors, and unplanned adverse outcomes.

EP23EO **Unit- or clinic-level patient satisfaction data (related to nursing care) outperform the mean or median of the national database used.**

IE

> ▸ Provide 8 quarters of inpatient, pediatric, and ambulatory/outpatient patient satisfaction data at the unit- or clinic-level collected within the previous 30 months before documentation submission. Select and report data for four of the nine categories listed below.
>
> 1. Patient engagement/patient-centered care
> 2. Care coordination
> 3. Safety
> 4. Service recovery (may be ambulatory)
> 5. Courtesy and respect
> 6. Responsiveness
> 7. Patient education
> 8. Pain
> 9. Careful listening
>
> *Note: Pediatric and ambulatory patient satisfaction data are required for organizations with these services in place.*

See *Addendum* on page 109 in the *2014 Magnet® Application Manual* for ambulatory data requirements.

IV. NEW KNOWLEDGE, INNOVATIONS & IMPROVEMENTS (NK)

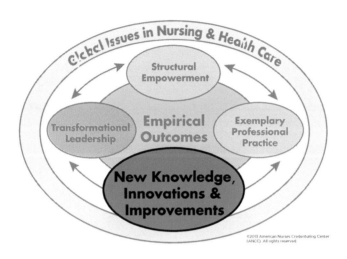

Forces of Magnetism:

▸ Quality of Care: Research and Evidence-Based Practice

▸ Quality Improvement

Magnet®-recognized organizations conscientiously integrate evidence-based practice and research into clinical and operational processes. Nurses are educated about evidence-based practice and research, enabling them to appropriately explore the safest and best practices for their patients and practice environment and to generate new knowledge. Published research is systematically evaluated and used. Nurses serve on the board that reviews proposals for research, and knowledge gained through research is disseminated to the community of nurses.

Organizations achieving Magnet recognition have established evolving programs related to evidence-based practices and research programs. Infrastructures and resources are in place to support the advancement of evidence-based practices and research in all clinical settings. Targets for research productivity are set with participation and leadership from nurses in a multitude of research activities within the framework of the practice site.

Innovations in patient care, nursing, and the practice environment are the hallmark of organizations receiving Magnet recognition. Establishing new ways of achieving high-quality, effective, and efficient care is the outcome of transformational leadership, empowering structures and processes, and exemplary professional practice in nursing.

Sources of Evidence

RESEARCH

NK1EO   **The organization supports the advancement of nursing research.** Provide one completed IRB-approved nursing research study. Use format presented on thefollowing page.

Introduction

▸ Research question and hypothesis

▸ Study rationale

▸ Literature review (two pages maximum)

Participants

▸ Nurse(s) at the organization who is (are) the principal investigator(s) (PI or co-PI) involved in the conduct of the study

Methods

▸ Study design

▸ Study timeline

  ▸▸ Start date

  ▸▸ Completed date

▸ IRB approval date: full committee/expedited review/exempt

▸ Research sample (study participants and sample size, sampling plan)

▸ Data collection methods

Results

▸ Results of data analysis (quantitative) or findings (qualitative); must have occurred within the four (4) years before documentation submission

Discussion

▸ Summary of key findings

▸ Analysis of the findings

▸ Implications of the findings

Note: For system applications, one completed nursing research study must be presented for each organization; if a combined study is presented, clear participation by each organization must be evident and outcome data must show an impact for each organization.

NK2   **Nurses disseminate the organization's nursing research findings to internal and external audiences.**

> ▸ Provide one example, with supporting evidence, of how clinical nurses disseminated to internal audiences knowledge obtained through the organization's nursing research.

AND

> ▸ Provide one example, with supporting evidence, of how clinical nurses disseminated to external audiences knowledge obtained through the organization's nursing research.

EVIDENCE-BASED PRACTICE

NK3   **Clinical nurses evaluate and use evidence-based findings in their practice.**

> ▸ Provide one example, with supporting evidence, of how clinical nurses used evidence-based findings to implement a practice new to the organization.

AND

> ▸ Provide one example, with supporting evidence, of how clinical nurses used evidence-based findings to revise an existing practice to improve care.

INNOVATION

NK4EO **Innovation in nursing is supported and encouraged.**

> ▸ Provide two examples, with supporting evidence, of an improvement that resulted from an innovation in nursing. Supporting evidence must be submitted in the form of a graph with a data table that clearly displays the data.

NK5EO **Nurses are involved with the design and implementation of technology to enhance the patient experience and nursing practice.**

- ▸ Provide one example, with supporting evidence, of an improvement that occurred due to a change in nursing practice resulting from clinical nurses' involvement with design and implementation of technology. Supporting evidence must be submitted in the form of a graph with a data table that clearly displays the data.

AND

- ▸ Provide one example, with supporting evidence, of an improvement in the patient experience that resulted from clinical nurses' involvement with design and implementation of technology. Supporting evidence must be submitted in the form of a graph with a data table that clearly displays the data.

NK6EO **Nurses are involved in the design and implementation of work flow improvements and space design to enhance nursing practice.**

- ▸ Provide one example, with supporting evidence, of nurse involvement in the design and implementation of work flow that resulted in operational improvement, waste reduction, or clinical efficiency. Supporting evidence must be submitted in the form of a graph with a data table that clearly displays the data.

OR

- ▸ Provide one example, with supporting evidence, of nurse involvement in the design and implementation of work space that resulted in operational improvement, waste reduction, or clinical efficiency. Supporting evidence must be submitted in the form of a graph with a data table that clearly displays the data.

V. EMPIRICAL OUTCOMES (EO)

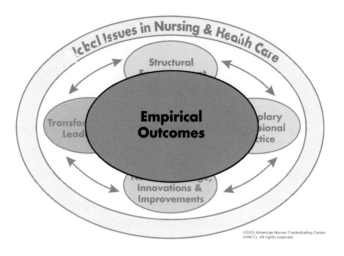

Forces of Magnetism:

▸ Quality Care

Nursing makes an essential contribution to patient, nursing workforce, organizational, and consumer outcomes. The empirical measurement of quality outcomes related to nursing leadership and clinical practice in Magnet-recognized organizations is imperative.

Throughout the *2014 Magnet® Application Manual*, in each of the other model components, the Empirical Outcomes are requested as Sources of Evidence.

Empirical Outcomes Presentation Requirements: SE3EO, EP3EO, EP22EO, EP23EO, NK1EO Only

The EOs for nursing certification (SE3EO), nurse (RN) satisfaction (EP3EO), nurse-sensitive clinical indicators (EP22EO), patient satisfaction (EP23EO), and nursing research (NK1EO) must be presented in the required format as outlined in the Sources of Evidence on the page number(s) listed below.

▸ SE3EO—page 16

▸ EP3EO—pages 24–25

▸ EP22EO—pages 32–33

▸ EP23EO—page 34

▸ NK1EO—page 36

Empirical Outcomes Presentation Requirements: All Others

For all other Empirical Outcomes, narratives must be presented using the following format:

Background/Problem
▸ Provide relevant background information
▸ Describe the problem(s) that exist(s) in the organization

Goal Statement(s)
▸ State the goal(s), that is the desired improvement(s)/change(s)/result(s)
▸ Identify the measure(s) selected to demonstrate the improvement(s)/change(s)/result(s) (i.e., hours, errors, incidents, satisfaction, indicators)

Description of the Intervention/Initiative/Activity(ies)
▸ Describe the action(s) that had an impact on the problem(s) and resulted in achievement of the goal(s)
  ▸▸ Include where the intervention(s)/initiative(s) occurred (e.g., unit, department, product line, organization)
  ▸▸ Include the date(s) when the intervention(s)/initiative(s) took place (timeline)
▸ The intervention(s)/initiative(s) must have occurred within the 30 months prior to documentation submission

Participants

▸ List the participants involved

▸ Include name, discipline, title, and department

Outcome(s)

▸ Demonstrate achievement of the desired improvement(s)/
change(s)/result(s) with data displayed in a clearly labeled
graph(s) with data table(s)

  ▸▸ Trended data must be displayed to show change(s)/
  improvement(s)/result(s); At a minimum, three (3) post-
  intervention data points must be provided to demonstrate a trend

  ▸▸ The selected measure(s) must correlate with the desired goal(s)

  ▸▸ Pre-intervention/initiative data and post-intervention/
  initiative data must:

    ▷ Use the same measure to demonstrate the effect of the
    intervention/initiative

    ▷ Be clearly identified with dates on the graph and data
    table

  ▸▸ The intervention time frame/date(s) must be clearly identified on
  the graph and data table

Empirical Outcomes: Data Display Requirements

Display of data using graphs and charts is an excellent way to illustrate
outcomes; therefore, a table and graph is required for each Empirical
Outcome.

Glossary

accountability

The ethical concept of being answerable or responsible for one's actions. In nursing, personal accountability is the responsibility nurses have to themselves and to patients, and public accountability is the responsibility nurses have to their employers and to society in general. "The primary goals of professional accountability in nursing are to maintain high standards of care and to protect the patient from harm. All nurses are accountable for the proper use of their knowledge and skills in the provision of care" (Farquharson, 2004, pp. 311–312).

acute care organization

A healthcare organization in which care is delivered to hospitalized patients.

advanced practice registered nurse (APRN)

A registered nurse who has met advanced educational and clinical practice requirements beyond the 2 to 4 years of basic nursing education required of all RNs. Under this umbrella are four principal types of APRNs: nurse practitioners, certified nurse midwives, clinical nurse specialists, and certified registered nurse anesthetists.

ambulatory/outpatient facility

A healthcare facility in which people, typically other than inpatients, visit healthcare providers for intervention and/or health counseling.

autonomy

Refers to clinical autonomy, organizational autonomy, and control over nursing practice.

care coordination

Care coordination is the extent to which patient care services are coordinated across people, functions, activities, and sites over time so as to maximize the value of services delivered to patients. Care coordination encompasses a set of practitioner behaviors and information systems intended to bring together health services, patient needs, and streams of information to facilitate the delivery of care (Institute of Medicine, 2004, p. 47).

care delivery system

A system for the delivery of care that delineates the nurses' authority and accountability for clinical decision-making and outcomes. The care delivery system is integrated with the professional practice model and promotes continuous, consistent, efficient, and accountable nursing care. The care delivery system is adapted to regulatory considerations and describes the context of care, the manner in which care is delivered, the skill set required, and expected outcomes of care.

certification

"A process by which a state regulatory body or a nongovernmental agency or association certifies that an individual licensed to practice a profession has met certain predetermined standards specified by that profession for specialty practice. Its purpose is to assure various publics that an individual has mastered a body of knowledge and acquired skills in a particular specialty. Title protection is granted to persons who have met the predetermined qualifications. Those without the title may perform the services of the profession or occupation but may not use the title" (ANCC, 2012). Certifications for ability to perform clinical interventions (e.g., Advanced Cardiac Life Support [ACLS], Basic Life Support [BLS], Neonatal Resuscitation Program [NRP], Pediatric Advanced Life Support [PALS]) are not included.

change

To undergo transformation, transition, or substitution (Merriam-Webster, 2013).

chief nursing officer (CNO)

The highest-level nurse with ultimate responsibility for all nursing practice within the organization.

clinical autonomy

Refers to the authority and freedom of nurses to make nursing care decisions (within the full scope of their practice) in the clinical care of patients within interprofessional practice environments (Weston, 2008).

clinical nurse

The registered nurse who spends the majority of his or her time providing direct patient care.

clinical practice

"Classification of nursing phenomena, nursing actions, and nursing outcomes that describes nursing practice" (Coenen, 2003).

community healthcare outreach

Organized action intended to provide outreach and cultural linkages between communities and delivery systems; reduce costs by providing health education, screening, detection, and basic emergency care; and improve quality by contributing to patient-provider communication, continuity of care, and consumer protection (adapted from Witmer, Seifer, Finocchio, Leslie, O'Neil, et al., 1995).

continuing nursing education (CNE) activities

Those learning activities intended to build upon the educational and experimental bases of an individual for the enhancement of practice, education, administration, research, or theory development, to the end of improving the health of the public (*ANCC Primary Application Accreditation Manual for Providers and Approvers*, ANCC, 2013).

continuing professional development (CPD)

Continuing professional development includes components of continuing education but has a broader focus and allows "health professionals to tailor the learning process, setting, and curriculum to their needs." The term CPD signals "the importance of multifaceted, lifelong learning in the lives of all health professionals" and recognizes that opportunities for learning stretch "from the classroom to the point of care." In a CPD system, individual practitioners have the flexibility to control and design their own learning (Institute of Medicine, 2010, p. 5).

control over nursing practice

Refers to the authority and freedom of nurses to engage in nursing practice decision-making (within the full scope of their practice) that includes organizational structures, governance, rules, policies, and operations (Weston, 2008).

efficiency

Avoiding waste, including waste of equipment, supplies, ideas, and energy (Institute of Medicine, 2001, p. 223).

evidence-based practice

The conscientious use/integration of the best research evidence with clinical expertise and patient preferences in nursing practice (adapted from Sackett et al., 2000). Evidence-based practice is a science-to-service model of engagement of critical thinking to apply research-based evidence (scientific knowledge) and practice-based evidence (art of nursing) within the context of patient values to deliver quality, cost-sensitive care. It is distinguished from practice-based evidence, a practice-to-science model in which data are derived from interventions thought to be effective but for which empirical evidence is lacking.

family

The basic unit in society traditionally consisting of two parents rearing their children; also, any of various social units differing from but regarded as equivalent to the traditional family (Merriam-Webster, 2013).

fundamentals of quality nursing care

1. The Nursing Professional Practice Model illustrates the alignment and integration of nursing practice with the mission, vision, philosophy, and values of the organization.

2. Nursing leadership develops a strong vision and well-articulated philosophy that supports and promotes high standards for nursing practice.

3. Nurses are clinically competent.

4. Nurses incorporate evidence-based findings and standards into the delivery of patient care.

5. Nurses partner with patients and families to diagnose, plan, and deliver individualized patient-centered care.

6. A culture of safety is promoted in the nurse work environment.

7. Nurses participate in the surveillance, reporting, and evaluation of continuous quality improvement.

influence

Actions that either directly or indirectly cause a change in the behavior and/or attitudes of another individual or group. The primary effect of leadership (Shortell & Kaluzny, 2000, p. 461).

innovation

"Innovation in service delivery and organization [is] a novel set of behaviors, routines, and ways of working that are directed at improving health outcomes, administrative efficiency, cost effectiveness, or users' experience and that are implemented by planned and coordinated actions" (Greenhalgh, 2004).

Institutional Review Board (IRB)

An independent committee composed of scientific, nonscientific, and nonaffiliated members that is established (according to U.S. federal regulations) to review, approve, and monitor research involving humans as participants, and to approve the initiation of and conduct periodic review of such research. The term includes but is not limited to Institutional Review Boards, Investigational Review Boards, Central Review Boards, Independent Review Boards, and Cooperative Research Boards (U.S. Department of Health and Human Services, n.d., [45 CFR §46.402(g)] [21 CFR §50.3(i)]).

interdisciplinary

"Reliant on the overlapping skills and knowledge of each team member and discipline; resulting in synergistic effects in which outcomes are improved and more comprehensive than the simple aggregation of any team member's individual efforts" (American Nurses Association, 2010, p. 66).

interprofessional

"Reliant on the overlapping skills and knowledge of each team member and discipline, resulting in synergistic effects in which outcomes are improved and more comprehensive than the simple aggregation of any team member's individual efforts" (American Nurses Association, 2010, p. 66). Examples of interprofessional decision-making groups may include but are not restricted to shared governance committees or project, process improvement, or product selection teams.

interprofessional collaborative practice

"Occurs when multiple health workers from different professional backgrounds provide comprehensive services by working with patients, their families, caregivers, and communities to deliver the highest quality of care across settings. Practice includes both clinical and non-clinical health-related work, such as diagnosis, treatment, surveillance, health communications, management and sanitation engineering" (WHO Study Group on Interprofessional Education & Collaborative Practice, 2010).

mentor

"An experienced nurse who has developed expertise and can be a strong force in shaping a nurse's identity as a professional" (Anthony, 2006, p. 73). Mentoring can include providing information, advice, support, and ideas. Typically, mentors and mentees have a long-lasting relationship.

mission

A statement of the good or benefit the healthcare organization intends to contribute, couched in terms of an identified community, a set of services, and a specific level of cost or finance (Griffith & White, 2002, p. 679).

new graduate

A nurse who has completed his or her nursing education and is in the first year of employment as a registered or licensed professional nurse. New graduates are generally novice nurses who have limited clinical experience and require orientation, guidance, mentorship, and safe learning environments to transition into beginning nursing practice. (Benner, Tanner, Chesla, 2009).

nurse leaders

Nurse leaders with line authority over multiple units that have RNs working clinically and nurse leaders who are positioned on the organizational chart between the nurse manager and the chief nursing officer. Includes nurse educators.

nurse managers

Registered nurses with 24-hour/7-day accountability for the supervision of all registered nurses and other healthcare providers who deliver nursing care in an inpatient or outpatient area. The nurse manager is typically responsible for recruitment and retention, performance review, and professional development; is involved in the budget formulation process and quality outcomes; and helps plan for, organize, and lead the delivery of nursing care for a designated patient care area.

Nurse Practice Act

The basic enabling law in states and territories within the United States for licensure and definition of nursing practice in the jurisdiction of the legislative body establishing the act. It defines who may practice nursing and, to some extent, how nursing will be practiced in the jurisdiction.

nurse (RN) satisfaction

Job satisfaction expressed by nurses working in hospital settings as determined by scaled responses to a uniform series of questions designed to elicit nursing staff attitudes toward specific aspects of their employment situation.

nurse-sensitive clinical indicators

"Measures and indicators that reflect the impact of nursing actions on outcomes" (American Nurses Association, 2009, p. 25).

nursing practice

Nursing practice encompasses autonomous and collaborative care of individuals of all ages, families, groups and communities, sick or well, and in all settings. Nursing includes the promotion of health, prevention of illness, and the care of ill, disabled, and dying people. Advocacy, promotion of a safe environment, research, participation in shaping health policy and in patient and health systems management, and education are also key nursing roles (Coenen, 2003).

nursing research

"Systematic inquiry that uses disciplined methods to answer questions or solve problems. The ultimate goal of research is to develop, refine, and expand knowledge" (Polit & Beck, 2012).

organization

A stand-alone structure within an entity; the term can be used interchangeably with setting where appropriate or necessary.

organizational autonomy

Refers to the authority and the freedom of a nurse to be involved in broader unit, service line, organization, or system decision-making processes pertaining to patient care, policies and procedures, and work environment (Weston, 2008).

outcomes

Quantitative and qualitative evidence related to the impact of structure and process on the patient, nursing workforce, organization, and consumer. These outcomes are dynamic and measurable and may be reported at an individual unit, department, population, or organizational level. Donabedian defined outcomes as the "changes (desirable or undesirable) in individuals and populations that can be attributed to health care" (Donabedian, 2003, p. 46).

patient

A healthcare consumer across the variety of settings; he or she might variously be called a patient, client, or resident.

patient satisfaction

Patient opinion of the care received during the hospital stay or in ambulatory/outpatient services, as determined by scaled responses to a uniform series of questions designed to elicit patient views about global aspects of care.

peer review

Peer-provided components of an annual evaluation or performance appraisal by which registered nurses assess and judge the performance of professional peers (i.e., registered nurses with similar roles and education, clinical expertise, and level of licensure) against established practice and organizational standards. The peer review process stimulates professionalism through increased accountability and promotes self-regulation of practice.

performance gap

Deficiencies in the performance of an organization. Recognition of this gap begins the initial stage in the change process within organizations (Shortell & Kaluzny, 2000, p. 464).

preceptor

"A skilled practitioner or faculty member who supervises students in a clinical setting to allow practical experience with patients" (Myrick & Yonge, 2005, p. 4).

pressure ulcer

Any lesion caused by pressure resulting in damage of underlying tissues. Other terms used to indicate this condition include bed sores and decubitus ulcers.

process

The actions involving the delivery of nursing and healthcare services to patients, including practices that are safe and ethical, autonomous, evidence-based, and focused on quality improvement. Donabedian defined process as the activities constituting health care, "including diagnosis, treatment, rehabilitation, prevention, and patient education—usually carried out by professional personnel, but also including other contributions to care, particularly by patients and their families" (Donabedian, 2003, p. 46).

professional nurse practice environment

A system that empowers nurses by providing them with increased opportunities for autonomy, accountability, and control over the care they provide and the environment in which they deliver that care (Zelauskas & Howes, 1992).

professional organization

Professional bodies, including in nursing, that may be known as organizations, associations, or societies, and that usually have the purpose of advancing a profession and protecting the public interest. It is an organization whose members belong to a particular profession that sets requirements and standards for entry into and maintaining membership in that profession (USLegal.com, 2013).

professional practice model

The driving force of nursing care; a schematic description of a theory, phenomenon, or system that depicts how nurses practice, collaborate, communicate, and develop professionally to provide the highest-quality care for those served by the organization (e.g., patients, families, communities). Professional practice models illustrate the alignment and integration of nursing practice with the mission, vision, and values that nursing has adopted.

quality improvement (QI)

"Systematic, data-guided activities designed to bring about immediate improvement in healthcare delivery in particular settings" (Lynn et al., 2007, p. 667).

registered nurse (RN)

A nurse in the United States who holds state board licensure as a registered nurse or any new graduate or foreign nurse graduate who is awaiting state board examination results and is employed by a healthcare organization with responsibilities of an RN. In other countries, this individual will have registered with the appropriate regulatory body.

research

A systematic investigation, including research development, testing, and evaluation, designed to develop or contribute to generalizable knowledge (U.S. Department of Health and Human Services, n.d., [45 CFR §46.102(d)] [21 CFR §50.3(k)] [21 CFR §312.3]). Research is distinguished from research utilization, the process of synthesizing, disseminating, and using research-generated knowledge to make an impact on, or a change in, the existing practices in society (Burns & Grove, 2005, p. 750).

shared leadership/participative decision-making

A model in which nurses are formally organized to make decisions about clinical practice standards, quality improvement, staff and professional development, and research.

strategic plan

A plan resulting from a process of "reviewing the mission, environmental surveillance, and previous planning decisions used to establish major goals and nonrecurring resource allocation decisions" (Griffith & White, 2002, p. 683).

structure

The characteristics of the organization and the healthcare system, including leadership, availability of resources, and professional practice models. Donabedian defined structure as the conditions under which care is provided, including material resources, human resources, and organizational characteristics "such as the organization of the medical and nursing staffs, the presence of teaching and research functions, kinds of supervision and performance review, and methods of paying for care" (Donabedian, 2003, p. 46).

transformational leadership

Transformational leaders are those who stimulate and inspire followers to both achieve extraordinary outcomes and, in the process, develop their own leadership capacity. They help followers grow and develop into leaders by responding to individual followers' needs by empowering them and by aligning the objectives and goals of the individual followers, the leader, the group, and the larger organization. Transformational leaders do more with followers and colleagues than set up simple exchanges or agreements—they behave in ways to achieve superior results by employing one or more of the four core components of transformational leadership, which are referred to as the 4 I's:

1. **Idealized Influence (II)**—Leaders serve as a role model for followers; they exhibit high ethical behavior, instill pride, and gain respect and trust. Followers tend to identify with their leaders and desire to emulate them; leaders are perceived by their followers as having extraordinary capabilities, persistence, and determination.

2. **Inspirational Motivation (IM)**—The degree to which the leader articulates a vision that is appealing, motivating, and inspiring to followers. Leaders with inspirational motivation communicate optimism about future goals, provide meaning for the task at hand, and challenge followers with high standards. The visionary aspects of leadership are supported by communication skills that make the vision understandable, precise, powerful, and engaging. The followers are

willing to invest more effort in their tasks because they are encouraged and optimistic about the shared vision and goals.

3. **Intellectual Stimulation (IS)**—The degree to which leaders challenge assumptions, take risks, and stimulate and solicit followers' ideas. Transformational leaders encourage followers to be innovative and creative by questioning assumptions, by reframing problems, and by challenging them to approach old situations in new ways.

4. **Individualized Consideration (IC)**—The degree to which the leader attends to each follower's needs for achievement and growth, acts as a mentor or coach to the follower, and listens to the follower's concerns and needs. The leader provides empathy and support, keeps communication open, and places challenges before the followers. IC also encompasses the need for respect and celebrates the individual contribution that each follower makes to the team (Bass & Riggio, 2006).

turnover

Number of employees who resigned, retired, expired, or were terminated divided by the number employed during the same period.

vacancy rate

Calculated as 1 minus full-time equivalents (FTEs)/whole-time equivalents (WTEs) employed divided by FTEs/WTEs budgeted times 100.

values statement

An expansion of the mission that expresses basic rules of acceptable conduct, such as respect for human dignity or acceptance of equality (Griffith & White, 2002, p. 684).

vision statement

An expansion of the mission that expresses intentions, philosophy, and organizational self-image (Griffith & White, 2002, p. 684).

work flow

Progression of steps (tasks, events, interactions) that compose a work process, involve two or more people, and create or add value to the organization's activities. In a sequential work flow, each step is dependent on occurrence of the previous step; in a parallel work flow, two or more steps can occur concurrently.

References

American Hospital Association. (2013). *Fast facts on US hospitals* [last updated January 3, 2013]. Retrieved March 27, 2013, from http://www.aha.org/aha/resource-center/Statistics-and-Studies/fast-facts.html.

American Nurses Association. (1979). *The study of credentialing in nursing: A new approach* (Vol. I, Report of the Committee). Kansas City, MO: Author.

American Nurses Association. (2001). *ANA's bill of rights for registered nurses.* Washington, DC: Author.

American Nurses Association. (2001b). *Code of ethics for nurses, with interpretive statements.* Silver Spring, MD: Author.

American Nurses Credentialing Center. (2004). *Magnet Recognition Program: Application Manual 2005.* Silver Spring, MD: Author.

American Nurses Credentialing Center. (2008). *Magnet Recognition Program: Application Manual 2008.* Silver Spring, MD: Author.

American Nurses Association. (2009). *Nursing administration: Scope and standards of practice* (2nd ed.). Silver Spring, MD: Author.

American Nurses Association. (2010). *Nursing professional development: Scope and standards of practice.* Silver Spring, MD: Author.

American Nurses Association. (2010). *Nursing: Scope and standards of practice* (2nd ed.). Silver Spring, MD: Author.

American Nurses Association. (2012). *ANA's principles for nurse staffing* (2nd ed.). Silver Spring, MD: Author.

Anthony, M. K. (2006). Professional practice and career development. In D. L. Huber (Ed.), *Leadership and nursing care management* (3rd ed.; pp. 61–81). Philadelphia, PA: Saunders Elsevier.

Bass, B. M., & Riggio, R. E. (2006). *Transformational leadership* (2nd ed.; p. 1–7). Mahwah, NJ: Lawrence Erlbaum Associates, Inc.

Benner, P. (1982). From novice to expert. *American Journal of Nursing*, 82(3), 402–407.

Benner, P., Tanner, C., & Chesla, C. (2009). *Expertise in nursing practice: caring, clinical judgment, and ethics* (2nd ed). New York: Springer Publishing.

Burns, J. (1978). *Leadership.* New York: Harper & Row.

Burns, N., & Grove, S. K. (2005). *The practice of nursing research: Conduct, critique, and utilization* (5th ed.). St. Louis, MO: Elsevier.

BusinessDictionary.com (2013). Workflow. Retrieved March 27, 2013, from http://www.businessdictionary.com/definition/workflow.html#ixzz2DdLLYWCO.

Coenen, A. (2003). The international classification for nursing practice (ICNP®) programme: Advancing a unifying framework for nursing. *The Online Journal of Issues in Nursing*, 8(2). Retrieved June 25, 2013, from http://www.nursingworld.org/MainMenuCategories/ANAMarketplace/ANAPeriodicals/OJIN/TableofContents/Volume82003/No2May2003/ArticlesPreviousTopics/TheInternationalClassificationforNursingPractice.html.

Dictionary.com. (2013). Enculturation. Retrieved June 25, 2013, from http://dictionary.reference.com/browse/enculturation?s=t.

Donabedian, A. (1980). *The definition of quality and approaches to its assessment.* Ann Arbor, MI: Health Administration Press.

Donabedian, A. (2003). *An introduction to quality assurance in health care.* New York: Oxford University Press.

Dunham-Taylor, J. (2000). Nurse executive transformational leadership found in participative organizations. *Journal of Nursing Administration*, 30(5), 241–250.

Farquharson, J. M. (2004). Liability of the nurse manager. In T. D. Aiken (Ed.), *Legal, ethical, and political issues in nursing* (2nd ed.; pp. 311–336). Philadelphia, PA: F.A. Davis Company.

Greenhalgh, T. (2004). Diffusion of innovations in service organizations: Systematic review and recommendations. *The Milbank Quarterly, 82,* 581–629.

Griffith, J. R., & White, K. R. (2002). *The well-managed healthcare organization* (5th ed.). Chicago: Health Administration Press.

Institute of Medicine. (2000). *To err is human: Building a safer health system.* Washington, DC: The National Academies Press.

Institute of Medicine. (2003). *Health professions education: A bridge to quality.* Washington, DC: The National Academies Press.

Institute of Medicine. (2004). *Patient safety: Achieving a new standard for care.* Washington, DC: The National Academies Press.

Institute of Medicine. (2004). *Report of a summit. The 1st annual crossing the quality chasm summit: A focus on committees.* Washington, DC: The National Academies Press.

Institute of Medicine. (2010). *Redesigning continuing education in the health professions.* Washington, DC: The National Academies Press.

Interprofessional Education Collaborative Expert Panel. (2011). *Core competencies for interprofessional collaborative practice: Report of an expert panel.* Washington, DC: Interprofessional Education Collaborative.

Lynn, J., Baily, M. A., Bottrell, M., et al. (2007). The ethics of using quality improvement methods in health care. *Annals of Internal Medicine, 146,* 666–673.

Merriam-Webster. (2013). Retrieved March 27, 2013, from http://www.merriam-webster.com.

Myrick, F., & Yonge, O. (2005). *Nursing preceptorship: Connecting practice and education*. Philadelphia, PA: Lippincott Williams & Wilkins.

National Research Council. (2004). *1st annual crossing the quality chasm summit: A focus on communities*. Washington, DC: The National Academies Press.

NTOCC Measures Work Group. (2008). *Transitions of care measures*. Washington, DC: National Transitions of Care Coalition. Retrieved March 27, 2013, from http://www.ntocc.org/Portals/0/PDF/Resources/TransitionsOfCare_Measures.pdf.

Polit, D., & Beck, C. T. (2012). *Nursing research: Generating and assessing evidence for nursing practice* (9th ed.). Philadelphia, PA: Lippincott Williams & Wilkins.

Reeves, S., & Lewin, S. (2004). Interprofessional collaboration in the hospital: Strategies and meanings. *Journal of Health Services Research & Policy*, 9(4), 218–225.

Sackett, D. L., Straus, S. E., Richardson, W. S., Rosenberg, W., & Haynes, R. B. (2000). *Evidence-based medicine: How to practice and teach EBM* (2nd ed.). Edinburgh: Churchill Livingstone.

Schaufeli, W., Salanova, M., González-Romá, V., & Bakker, A. (2002). The measurement of engagement and burnout: A two sample confirmatory factor analytic approach. *Journal of Happiness Studies*, 3(1), 71–92.

Scott, J., & Marshall, G. (Eds.). (2005). *A dictionary of sociology*. New York: Oxford University Press.

Tew, L. (2011). Human error management—Quality drives economic value. The Center for Error Management. Retrieved March 27, 2013, from http://manageerror.com/n_quality.htm.

The Beryl Institute. (2013). Defining patient experience. Retrieved March 27, 2013, from http://www.theberylinstitute.org/?page=DefiningPatientE xp&hhSearchTerms=definition+and+of+and+patient+and+experience.

Urden, L. D., & Monarch, K. (2002). The ANCC Magnet Recognition Program: Converting research findings into action. In M. L. McClure & A. S. Hinshaw (Eds.), *Magnet hospitals revisited: Attraction and retention of professional nurses* (pp. 103–116). Washington, DC: American Nurses Association.

USLegal.com. (2013). Professional association. Retrieved June 25, 2013, from http://definitions.uslegal.com/p/professional-association/.

U.S. Department of Health and Human Services. (n.d.). Code of Federal Regulations Title 45 Public Welfare Part 46: Protection of Human Subjects, Title 21 Food and Drugs Part 50: Protection of Human Subjects. Washington, DC: Author.

Weston, M. J. (2008). Defining control over nursing practice and autonomy. *Journal of Nursing Administration*, 38(9), 404–408.

WHO Study Group on Interprofessional Education and Collaborative Practice. (2010). *Framework for action on interprofessional education and collaborative practice.* Geneva, Switzerland: World Health Organization, Department of Human Resources for Health. Retrieved March 27, 2013, from http://www.who.int/hrh/resources/framework_action/en/.

Witmer, A., Seifer, S. D., Finocchio, L., Leslie, J., & O'Neil, E. H. (1995). Community health workers: Integral members of the health care work force. *American Journal of Public Health*, 85(8 Pt 1), 1055–1058. Retrieved March 27, 2013, from http://www.ncbi.nlm.nih.gov/pmc/ articles/PMC1615805/.

Zelauskas, B., & Howes, D. G. (1992). The effects of implementing a professional practice model. *Journal of Nursing Administration*, 22 (7/8), 18–23.

1. **Quality of nursing leadership**—Nursing leaders were perceived as knowledgeable, strong risk takers who followed an articulated philosophy in the day-to-day operations of the nursing department. Nursing leaders also conveyed a strong sense of advocacy and support on behalf of the staff.

   Expectations of a Magnet Organization 2005: Knowledgeable, strong, risk-taking nurse leaders follow a well-articulated, strategic, and visionary philosophy in the day-to-day operations of the nursing services. Nursing leaders at all levels of the organization convey a strong sense of advocacy and support for the staff and for the patient. (The results of quality leadership are evident in nursing practice at the patient's side.)

2. **Organizational structure**—Organizational structures were characterized as flat, rather than tall, and unit-based decision-making prevailed. Nursing departments were decentralized, with strong nursing representation evident in the organizational committee structure. The nursing leader served at the executive level of the organization, and the chief nursing officer reported to the chief executive officer.

   Expectations of a Magnet Organization 2005: Organizational structures are generally flat, rather than tall, and decentralized decision-making prevails. The organizational structure is dynamic and responsive to change. Strong nursing representation is evident in the organizational committee structure. Executive-level nursing leaders serve at the executive level of the organization. The CNO typically reports directly to the chief executive officer. The organization has a functioning and productive system of shared decision-making.

3. **Management style**—Hospital and nursing administrators were found to use a participative management style, incorporating feedback from staff at all levels of the organization. Feedback was characterized

as encouraged and valued. Nurses serving in leadership positions were visible, accessible, and committed to communicating effectively with staff.

Expectations of a Magnet Organization 2005: The healthcare organization and nursing leaders create an environment supporting participation. Feedback is encouraged and valued and is incorporated from the staff at all levels of the organization. Nurses serving in leadership positions are visible, accessible, and committed to communicating effectively with staff.

4. **Personnel policies and programs**—Salaries and benefits were characterized as competitive. Rotating shifts were minimized, and creative and flexible staffing models were used. Personnel policies were created with staff involvement, and important administrative and clinical promotional opportunities existed.

Expectations of a Magnet Organization 2005: Salaries and benefits are competitive. Creative and flexible staffing models that support a safe and healthy work environment are used. Personnel policies are created with direct-care nurse involvement. Important opportunities for professional growth exist in administrative and clinical tracks. Personnel policies and programs support professional nursing practice, work/life balance, and the delivery of quality care.

5. **Professional models of care**—Models of care were used that gave nurses the responsibility and authority for the delivery of patient care. Nurses were accountable for their own practice and were the coordinators of care.

Expectations of a Magnet Organization 2005: There are models of care that give nurses the responsibility and authority for the delivery of direct patient care. Nurses are accountable both for their own practice and for the coordination of care. The models of care (i.e., primary nursing, case management, family-centered, district, holistic) provide for the continuity of care across the continuum. The models take into consideration patients' unique needs and provide skilled nurses and adequate resources to accomplish desired outcomes.

6. **Quality of care**—Nurses perceived that they were providing high-quality care to their patients. Providing quality care was seen as an organizational priority as well, and nurses serving in leadership positions were viewed as responsible for developing the environment in which high-quality care could be provided.

   Expectations of a Magnet Organization 2005: Quality is the systematic driving force for nursing and the organization. Nurses serving in leadership positions are responsible for providing an environment that positively influences patient outcomes. The pervasive perception among nurses is that they provide high-quality care to patients/residents/clients.

7. **Quality improvement**—Quality improvement activities were viewed as educational. Staff nurses participated in the quality improvement process and perceived the process as one that improved the quality of care delivered within the organization.

   Expectations of a Magnet Organization 2005: The organization has structures and processes for the measurement of quality and programs for improving the quality of care and services within the organization.

8. **Consultation and resources**—Adequate consultation and other human resources were available. Knowledgeable experts, particularly advanced practice nurses, were available and consulted. In addition, peer support was given within and from outside the nursing division.

   Expectations of a Magnet Organization 2005: The healthcare organization provides adequate resources, support, and opportunities for use by experts, particularly advanced practice registered nurses. In addition, the organization promotes involvement of nurses in professional organizations and among peers in the community.

9. **Autonomy**—Nurses were permitted and expected to practice autonomously, consistent with professional standards. Independent judgment was expected to be exercised within the context of a multidisciplinary approach to patient care.

   Expectations of a Magnet Organization 2005: Autonomous nursing care is the ability of a nurse to assess and provide nursing actions as appropriate for patient care based on competence, professional expertise, and knowledge. The nurse is expected to practice autonomously, consistent with professional standards. Independent judgment is expected to be exercised within the context of interdisciplinary and multidisciplinary approaches to patient/resident/client care.

10. **Community and the hospital**—Hospitals that were best able to recruit and retain nurses also maintained a strong community presence. A community presence was seen in a variety of ongoing, long-term outreach programs. These outreach programs resulted in the hospital being perceived as a strong, positive, and productive corporate citizen.

Expectations of a Magnet Organization 2005: Relationships are established within and among all types of healthcare organizations and other community organizations, to develop strong partnerships that support improved patient outcomes and the health of the communities the nurses serve.

11. **Nurses as teachers**—Nurses were permitted and expected to incorporate teaching in all aspects of their practice. Teaching was one activity that reportedly gave nurses a great deal of professional satisfaction.

Expectations of a Magnet Organization 2005: Professional nurses are involved in educational activities within the organization and community. Students from a variety of academic programs are welcomed and supported in the organization; contractual arrangements are mutually beneficial. There is a development and mentoring program for staff preceptors for all levels of students (e.g., students, new graduates, experienced nurses). Staff in all positions serve as faculty and preceptors for students from a variety of academic programs. There is a patient education program that meets the diverse needs of patients in all the care settings of the organization.

12. **Image of nursing**—Nurses were viewed as integral to the hospital's ability to provide patient care services. The services provided by nurses were characterized as essential to other members of the healthcare team.

Expectations of a Magnet Organization 2005: The services provided by nurses are characterized as essential by other members of the healthcare team. Nurses are viewed as integral to the healthcare organization's ability to provide patient care. Nurses effectively influence system-wide processes.

13. **Interdisciplinary (interprofessional) relationships**—Interdisciplinary (interprofessional) relationships were characterized as positive. A sense of mutual respect was exhibited among all disciplines.

Expectations of a Magnet Organization 2005: Collaborative working relationships within and among the disciplines are valued. Mutual respect is based on the premise that all members of the healthcare team make essential and meaningful contributions in the achievement of clinical outcomes. Conflict management strategies are in place and are used effectively, when indicated.

14. **Professional development**—Strong emphasis was placed on orientation, in-service education, continuing education, formal education, and career development. Personal and professional growth and development were valued. In addition, opportunities for competency-based clinical advancement existed, along with the resources to maintain competency.

Expectations of a Magnet Organization 2005: The healthcare organization values and supports the personal and professional growth and development of staff. In addition to quality orientation and in-service education addressed earlier in Force 11, emphasis is placed on providing career development services. Programs that promote formal education, professional certification, and career development are evident. Competency-based clinical and leadership/management development is promoted, and adequate human and fiscal resources for all professional development programs are provided.

Sources: American Nurses Credentialing Center (2004, pp. 36–65), Urden and Monarch (2002, pp. 106–107).

66257310R00044

Made in the USA
Charleston, SC
13 January 2017